'This book is incredibly inspirational. A feel-good, call-to-action to be kind!'

—

David R. Hamilton, Ph.D., author and international speaker

'Kindness is the foundation for a happier world. This wonderful book is packed with inspiring and practical ways that we can all help to spread more ripples of kindness and happiness in our daily lives. Highly recommended.'

—

Dr Mark Williamson, director of Action for Happiness

'To me kindness is giving selflessly. It's to give with no expectation. A smile, a helping hand, a warm gesture … just because your heart desires to do a good deed for no other reason than to make someone happy. 52 Lives is amazing, selfless and truly wonderful.'

—

Gemma Oaten, actor

'*Kindness* is overflowing with inspiring messages to help us all remember the importance of being kind. Whether you're young or old, these are inspiring reminders of how we can make society better for all of us.'

—

Bullying UK, part of Family Lives

'I was always bought up to show loving kindness towards others. To help others, like 52 Lives does, is a selfless act. It doesn't cost anything to be kind and it can mean so much – a simple smile costs nothing.'

—

Duncan James, singer from Blue, actor and presenter

'In a world divided by terror and fear, I genuinely believe that kindness can bring us together. Jaime and the light she brings to this funny old planet is very much needed.'

—

Emily Coxhead, founder of *The Happy Newspaper*

For my three kind
little beating hearts,
Abbey, Max and Joseph

And for Greig, my
love and the kindest
person I know

Thorsons
An imprint of HarperCollins*Publishers*
1 London Bridge Street
London SE1 9GF

www.harpercollins.co.uk

First published by Thorsons 2017

10 9 8 7 6 5 4 3 2 1

Text © Jaime Thurston 2017

Illustrations © Debbie Powell 2017

Jaime Thurston asserts the moral right to
be identified as the author of this work

A catalogue record of this book is
available from the British Library

ISBN 978-0-00-825284-7

Printed and bound in Latvia

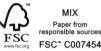

MIX
Paper from
responsible sources
www.fsc.org   **FSC™ C007454**

This book is produced from independently certified FSC™ paper
to ensure responsible forest management.

For more information visit: www.harpercollins.co.uk/green

FSC™ is a non-profit international
organisation established to promote the
responsible management of the world's
forests. Products carrying the FSC label
are independently certified to assure
consumers that they come from forests
that are managed to meet the social,
economic and ecological needs of
present and future generations, and
other controlled sources.

Find out more about HarperCollins
and the environment at
www.harpercollins.co.uk/green

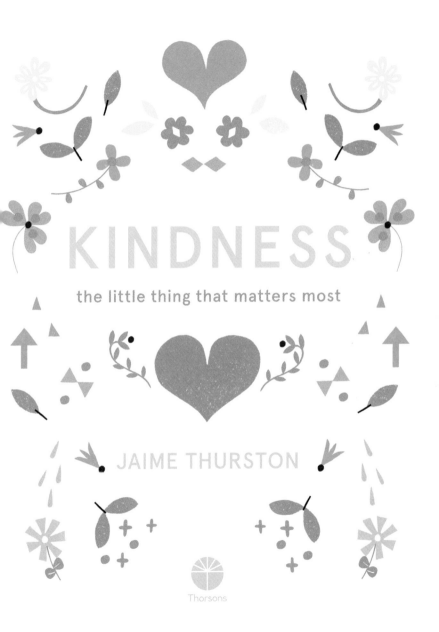

KINDNESS

the little thing that matters most

JAIME THURSTON

Thorsons

Contents

Foreword

David R. Hamilton, Ph.D., author of *The Five Side Effects of Kindness*

Kindness is the glue that holds society together. It is the essence of beauty. It brings smiles to faces, lightens our burdens, creates friendships, transforms people and situations. It can make a day memorable. It can be the answer to someone's prayers. This is how I see Jaime Thurston's work with 52 Lives. It is heart-warming to see how she makes a difference in so many people's lives.

And I mean heart-warming in two ways. First, in the sense that it makes us feel uplifted and inspired. Second, in that observing or learning about kindness does create a warming sensation in the heart. Kindness produces oxytocin and nitric oxide, two substances that directly affect our arteries, softening them, dilating them, reducing blood pressure, clearing them of free radicals, and increasing blood flow to the heart.

It's part of what social psychologist, Jonathan Haidt, calls 'elevation', which we feel when we're being kind, receiving kindness, or witnessing kindness. This also inspires us to pay kindnesses forward. This in turn sets in motion the well-known ripple effect of kindness, where one act touches many more lives than just the original recipient.

We are wired to be kind. It's our deepest nature. We have kindness genes that are some of the oldest in the human genome, at over 500 million years young. Looking out for each other is human nature.

I hope this book warms you and may your kindnesses in turn warm the hearts of many others. Of the different talked-about ways of changing the world for the better, I believe that kindness carries our best hope.

David

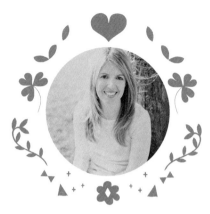

Introduction

'Urgently needed – rugs.' That was the message that started everything. I was searching online for second-hand furniture, when I came across the plea for help. It was a Wanted ad placed by a woman who sounded desperate. I emailed her and was heartbroken by what I learned. She needed the rugs to cover her broken floor so her young children wouldn't cut their feet. She was a single mum who had fled a horrifying domestic situation and was starting all over again with nothing. I wanted to help her, and I was sure that if others knew about her, they would want to help, too. So I spread the word among my friends and family, and household goods soon started pouring in.

I delivered everything to her one afternoon – piles of bedding, furniture, kitchenware, clothing, toys and some gift vouchers. I will never forget the look on her face when she opened the door. She was in complete shock that people she didn't even know would be willing to help her. This was a woman very much in need of kindness, and strangers helped her feel loved when she needed it the most.

I wanted to do more ... I wanted to do this every week. And so 52 Lives was born. It started life as a simple Facebook page I set up so my friends and family could help people, but over the weeks, months and years, it grew into a global community of people who wanted to spread kindness and help others.

Each week, we choose someone, somewhere in the world, in need of help, share their story on our website and social media pages, request what they need, and our supporters offer help. It's based on the premise that people are good and want to help one another – and that lots of good people working together can achieve amazing things.

52 Lives helps anyone, from anywhere, with anything; our only criterion is that the person is in need of kindness. In the few years since 52 Lives began, we have changed people's lives in such a wonderful variety of ways – from buying teeth for a man in Alabama to building a sensory shed for a toddler in south London who was losing her sight, making video messages for a young boy being bullied, supplying wheelchairs to children in China and the UK, and sending a little girl and her grandmother on a holiday after the death of the girl's mother.

Although we give people tangible help, the philosophy behind it goes much deeper than simply supplying goods or services. The people we help all say the same thing: that it wasn't the 'thing' we gave them that changed their life, it was the kindness ... the fact that complete strangers cared about them. The people we help are going through quite difficult times and when you're in those situations, a little bit of kindness can make all the difference in the world.

A homeless asylum seeker from London called Maria was a perfect example of this. I read about Maria in a newspaper and contacted the journalist who wrote the article to see if we could help. Maria was raped, had fallen pregnant and was homeless.

With just weeks until her baby was due, she was lost in the system and receiving very little help from social services because of issues with her paperwork. She was finally given a room in a shared house just before her baby was born, but she had nothing and nobody to help her. I set up an Amazon wishlist for Maria and filled it with everything I could think of that she might need to care for her baby. I was actually a little worried we might not be able to help her – I was aware asylum can be a controversial issue and I thought I might end the week having to buy all the goods on the list myself! But I shared it on the 52 Lives website and stood back and watched as every single item on the list was bought – within an hour. These gifts helped Maria enormously, but more importantly, she didn't feel alone any more. And this human connection is what changes lives. Not just for the person receiving but also the person giving. Kindness changes all of us.

David Hamilton, a best-selling author, doctor and expert in the science of kindness, has written so much about the benefits of being kind. Through his work and his books, he has managed to use science to explain what the rest of us perhaps knew intuitively but couldn't verbalise – kindness makes us feel good, mentally and physically. I am a big fan of David's and feel honoured to have his support for this book. Many of his facts and figures about the science of kindness are peppered throughout these pages.

The most important thing I think we can learn is that being kind doesn't have to be about making grand gestures, or spending a lot of money or setting up your own charity – that's not what changes the world. Doing something (doing anything) to help another human being is what changes the world. And so I have filled this book with 52 ideas for incorporating more kindness into your world, because kindness is essential for our collective well-being.

Whatever your political views, the last couple of years have been filled with turmoil and uncertainty. But we are not powerless. A famous anthropologist, Margaret Mead, once said: 'Never doubt that a small group of thoughtful, committed citizens can change the world; indeed, it's the only thing that ever has.' Her words sum up the whole philosophy of 52 Lives and the aim of this book. Our everyday actions determine the kind of world we live in; it's the little things that matter most. So let's choose kindness.

Give

KIND COMMENTS

01

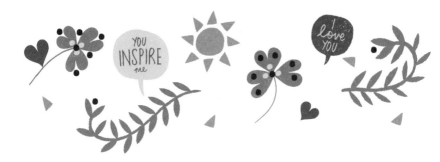

Unexpected kindness is a powerful thing. With just a few kind words, you can change someone's entire day.

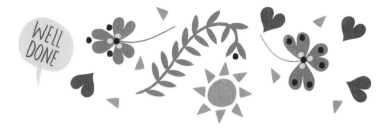

The people we care about the most are often the ones we forget to be kind to – we know they'll love us anyway and forgive any grumpiness. But one simple sentence can change everything. You have the power with every comment you make, every day, to help lift those around you – and yourself in the process. Don't underestimate the effect of a few kind words …

+ Tell your boss he or she inspires you
+ Tell your child you appreciate how hard they try
+ Tell your teacher they make coming to school fun
+ Tell your friends you love spending time with them
+ Tell your parents how much their support means to you
+ Tell your brother or sister you feel lucky to have them
+ Tell your partner they are the love of your life.

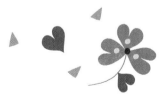

Be kind to
UNKIND PEOPLE

(they need it the most)

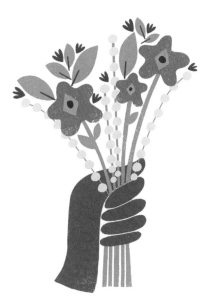

18 When someone is unkind to you, it's tempting to stoop to their level. But much like kindness breeds kindness, hate breeds hate.

18 KINDNESS – THE LITTLE THING THAT MATTERS MOST

It's the reason we often feel worse after an argument – being unkind, or being around unkindness, brings us down. If someone is being rude or angry, try to respond with kindness. It can change people's attitudes and help them see the world as a lovely place again. Choosing to fight unkindness with kindness will also have a positive effect on your own well-being, so you have nothing to lose!

' Being kind, receiving kindness or witnessing kindness makes us feel "elevated". It's the term psychologists use for the warm feeling we get. Studies show that elevation inspires people to be kind. So, when a person receives some kindness or even witnesses kindness, they feel elevated, and in turn, become extra kind themselves. Elevation is the feeling that causes kindness to be contagious. '

– *David R. Hamilton, Ph.D., from* The Five Side Effects of Kindness

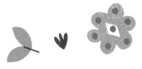

#02 – BE KIND TO UNKIND PEOPLE

03

Share
YOUR FOOD

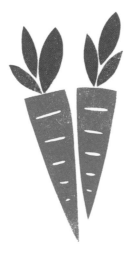

Next time you go shopping,
buy one extra thing at the
supermarket and donate it
to your local food bank.

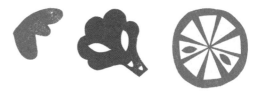

‘ I lie to my son. I tell him I've eaten during the day when I haven't. I barely have any money for food after bills and rent. So when he gets home from college, I just say I don't need to eat. But I can't live like that for ever. Without the food bank, I don't know what I would do. A friend had given me some shoes, and bits of clothing, but I didn't have food. I hope that one day I'll be able to pay back people's kindness. ’

— *Jenny, a single mum with disabilities who relies on food banks to survive*

Thousands of people rely on donations to feed their families. Feeding a hungry person is more than kindness – it's basic humanity. Giving one small tin or packet might seem insignificant, but they mean everything to those who receive them.

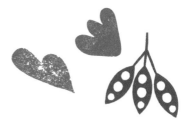

04

Do something
FOR NOTHING

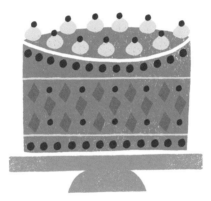

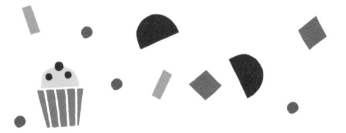

Sometimes what people need is assistance rather than things. Spread some kindness by donating a skill.

Donating in this way serves the dual purpose of fulfilling a practical need and making someone feel supported. Josh Coombes is a hairdresser who gives free haircuts to homeless people and founded a movement called 'Do Something For Nothing'. He says, 'Everyone has the power to do something for nothing. If everyone, in every city, did one thing for nothing, we could change the world.'

+ Cut someone's hair
+ Bake a cake
+ Mow a lawn
+ Help fill in a form
+ Mend someone's clothes
+ Do someone's taxes
+ Share your skill – teach someone what you know so they can pass on the kindness.

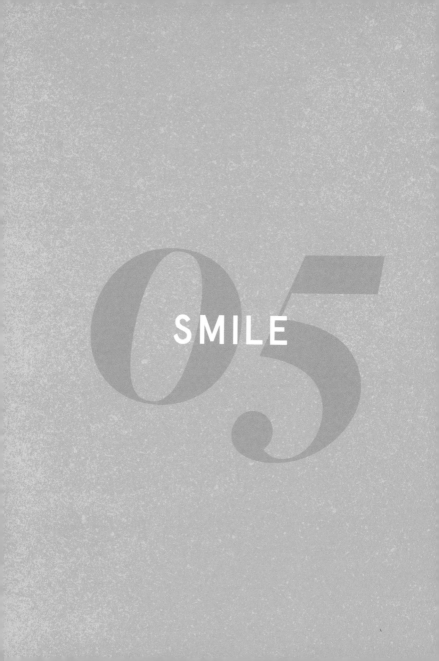

05

SMILE

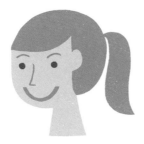

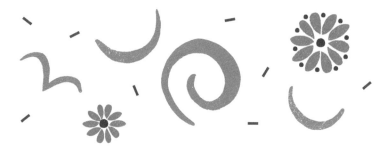

There's no such thing as
a small act of kindness –
even the tiniest gesture
has a ripple effect.

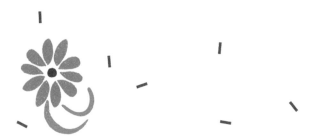

We don't tend to think of smiling as giving something to someone, but it is probably the most simple yet powerful thing we can do to spread kindness and happiness around the world. Not only does it lift another's mood – it's contagious!

In the brain, we have an interconnected network of cells known as the Mirror Neuron System (MNS for short). It causes us to mirror the facial expressions, body movements and gestures of other people. In the presence of someone expressing negative emotion, your MNS mirrors the movements of their facial muscles. So when they frown, you frown. On the up side, this same system gives all of us the power to spread smiles all over the world! So when you smile at someone, without them even realising it, their smile muscles will be stimulated.

— *David R. Hamilton, Ph.D.*

06

Switch off
AND CONNECT

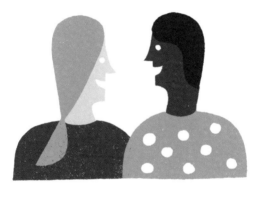

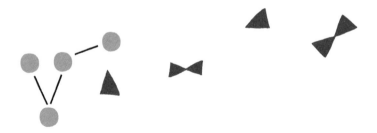

Face-to-face conversations allow us to truly connect as human beings and form deep, meaningful relationships.

We are more 'social' than ever online, but this can lead to a lack of real-life human connection – especially when we have access to an addictive virtual world in the palm of our hands.

The average phone user clicks, taps or swipes their phone 2,617 times a day during 76 different sessions, and stares at the screen for 145 minutes a day, according to a study by research company Dscout. However, it is real-life contact that human beings need. A University of Michigan study found that replacing face-to-face contact with emails, text messages and phone calls can double the risk of depression. But meeting our loved ones at least three times a week reduces this risk. Try to switch off your gadgets, look up and talk to people. Interacting in this way can help to alleviate depression and feelings of isolation, and ultimately makes us more kind. A smiley emoji is no replacement for the sound of a friend's laughter.

07

Send

KIND THOUGHTS

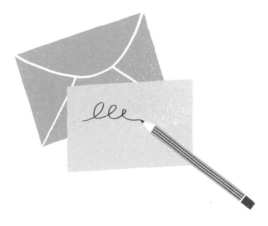

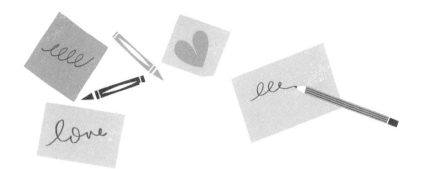

When someone is
struggling, knowing there

are people out there who
care can change everything.
It might even save their life.

The right words at the right time can change someone's life. If you know someone who is having a hard time, send a little note to let them know you're there. Write a letter, post a card or just send a quick email letting them know they are in your thoughts.

' I've kept every message I was sent from 52 Lives supporters and on my bad days – and there are bad days – I sit down and re-read them. The words from complete strangers are enough to lift my day. To know there are so many people out there who care really does make a difference. The gifts were wonderful, but honestly the messages meant more to me than the presents. '

— *Alyson has disabilities and is cared for full-time by her partner, Alan. 52 Lives supporters sent the couple gifts and messages.*

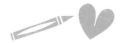

Give a gift to a
LOCAL SCHOOL

08

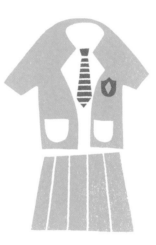

Your gesture will spread
so much kindness
and give happiness to
a child in need of help.

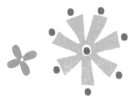

'We often see children coming to school without proper shoes to sit comfortably in for the day. When 52 Lives collected shoes and gift vouchers for our disadvantaged families, the response was, for many parents, overwhelming. They were truly touched at the kindness from complete strangers. It meant some of the children had their feet measured for the first time and shoes that fitted correctly and were comfortable.'

—*Hannah, a British schoolteacher whose class was helped by 52 Lives*

Contact your local school and ask how you can donate a book, toy, school shoes or a gift-card for school uniforms that can be passed on to someone who needs it. Many schools have welfare officers, who know which families in their school might be in need of help.

09

Pay for someone's
JOURNEY

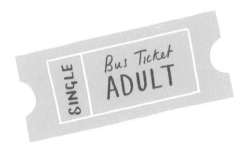

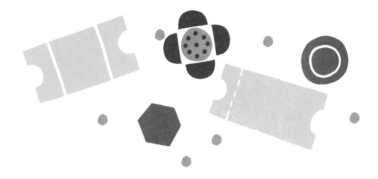

Altruism fosters a sense of connection. When we give something to someone, they feel closer to us, and we also feel closer to them.

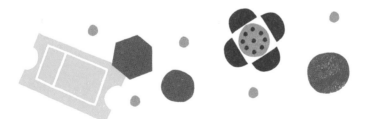

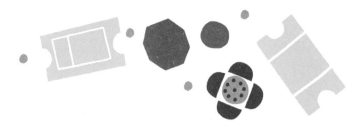

When you're out in the world and see someone struggling, see if you can help them on their way. Are they grappling to find change for the bus, or re-tapping a travel card that's not working? Step forward and offer help when you can. Being more conscious of the struggles of people around us – however small – means we can show kindness when people need it most. Something as simple as paying for someone's journey has the potential to turn around their whole day.

Psychologist Sonja Lyubomirsky, author of *The How of Happiness*, writes that being kind and generous leads us to perceive others more positively and more charitably, which in turn fosters a heightened sense of interdependence and cooperation in our social community.

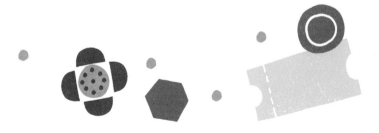

10

Remember where
YOU CAME FROM
(and where you are going)

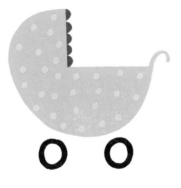

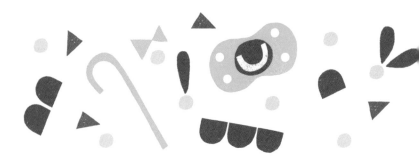

We are all at different

stages of the same journey,

and we're all in it together.

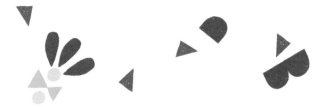

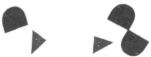

Try to be understanding of people at different stages of life – teenagers might seem disrespectful, parents with small children on your bus might seem annoying, and an older person in front of you might be walking a bit slowly. Perhaps that young person was you 20 years ago, and that pensioner will be you in the future?

" When my youngest grandchild was born, healthy and safe, I felt incredibly grateful, but I was also aware that a lot of babies were being born in less joyful circumstances. I decided to devote a year of my life to helping young families. As the year progressed, I learned that sometimes a small gesture can make a big difference. Of course that year has long passed, but it changed my life. I'm still "passing on" and I hope that along the way something I've done has made a difference. "

– Christine, a grandmother who helps change the lives of many families through 52 Lives

11

Be a seat

VIGILANTE

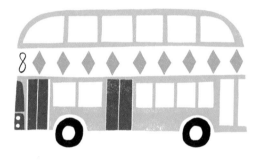

Sacrificing your seat
will help more than one

individual – you will be

helping to build a healthier,

kinder community.

If you feel able to stand up for a few stops on your bus or train, you don't need to wait for a disabled, elderly or pregnant person. Try being more conscious of those around you. Be kind to anyone you think might need the seat more than you. There may be a parent with young children, someone carrying heavy bags, or someone who just looks stressed and tired, who will appreciate your kind gesture. How lovely would the world be if we all did this?

A town in Pennsylvania called Roseto was put under the microscope after it was found that not a single person in the town under forty-five had died of heart disease in fifty years. Scientists descended on the town and eventually figured it out ... close community bonds were causing high levels of oxytocin (a cardio-protecting hormone) to flow, protecting the residents' hearts. It is known as the Roseto effect.

— *David R. Hamilton, Ph.D., from* The Five Side Effects of Kindness

12

APOLOGISE

Saying sorry does more
than simply remedy a
past mistake – it builds
a connection by showing
vulnerability and honesty.

58

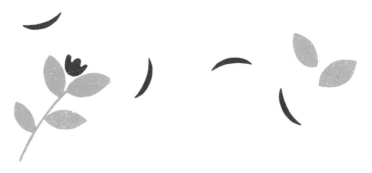

Everyone has bad days, and sometimes we take it out on people we don't even know. If in a moment of frustration or tiredness you find yourself doing this, be courageous and try to go back and apologise. I've returned to banks, shops and cafés lots of times to say sorry to people I was rude to and it made both me and the person I apologised to feel so much better! Finding the strength to apologise is especially important when it comes to our loved ones – the people we are closest to often bear the brunt of our negative emotions, but saying sorry will help to repair and rebuild.

The best apologies include accepting responsibility for what you did, and offering to make amends, according to research by Ohio State University. So when you apologise make it genuine by admitting you were wrong and avoid shifting the blame or making excuses – it's the difference between 'I'm sorry, I was wrong' and 'I'm sorry, but ...'

13

Be nice to parking
ATTENDANTS

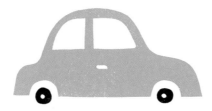

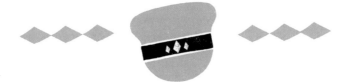

When we judge people
by their profession, we
cease to see them as
individuals. Try to override
assumptions and bias.

62

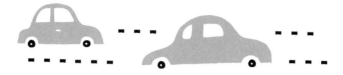

We often make judgements about people based on past experience, or things we've heard or read. Parking attendants are a good example of this. It seems to have become socially acceptable to be horrible to anyone working in this profession, simply for doing their job. Look for the people behind the profession – fellow human beings, all doing the best they can. And next time you see a parking attendant, smile and say hello!

' I get less abuse than I expected when I took this job – there have only been a couple of incidents where I've been threatened. It's mostly just people giving me a lot of bad attitude. It's not good, and I end up giving attitude back, even though I know I shouldn't. I understand why people get mad, but I'm just trying to work. '

— A parking attendant (who gave me a parking ticket!)

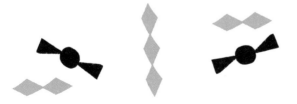

#13 – BE NICE TO PARKING ATTENDANTS

Speak

UP

14

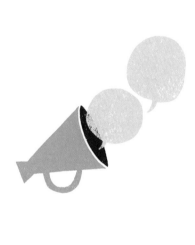

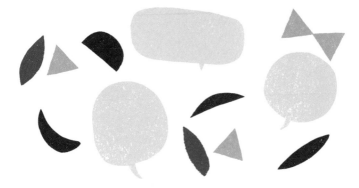

Be strong for those who
can't be, and be a voice
for those who need it.

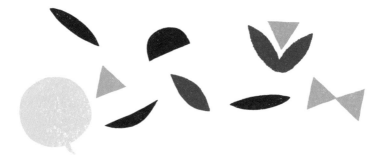

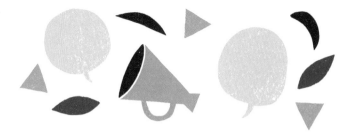

If you see someone being mistreated, whether it's at work, school or in your social group, speak up, let them know they aren't alone, or tell someone who can help. Irish statesman Edmund Burke's sentiment still rings true – when good people do nothing, evil triumphs. Don't do nothing.

' I lost all my self-confidence and couldn't face going outside. I'd always held my head high and been a leader, but after it happened I didn't even want to leave the house. Then messages came flooding in, one by one, from people all over the world. Because of everybody's kindness, I can walk outside again with my head held high and although I may not be such a leader now, I'm getting there with the support of everybody who has been kind to me. '

— *Toby, a 12-year-old boy who was bullied and beaten while onlookers filmed. Toby received hundreds of messages and gifts from 52 Lives supporters*

15

Share

GOOD NEWS

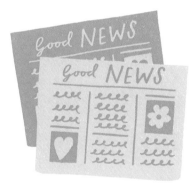

Sharing good news spreads
positivity, changes attitudes

70

and ultimately leads
to more people feeling
encouraged and happy.

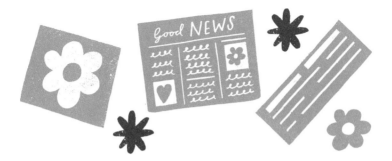

When you hear or read about something good, share it! All too often we share the scandalous, the shocking or the heartbreaking. There is so much good happening in the world. We just need to draw attention to it.

‘ In a world which can be very overwhelming, a world where we see nothing but terror and fear on our TV screens and on our phones ... it's easy to forget how much good stuff there actually is. Although we may not be able to change the whole world, we can have a positive impact on those around us. If more of us shared more positive news and created our own "happy news" with small acts of kindness incorporated into our daily lives, it would make the world (or a few people's worlds) a much happier place. ’

— *Emily Coxhead, founder of* The Happy News, *a newspaper and movement spreading happiness all over the world*

16

Stop comparing YOURSELF

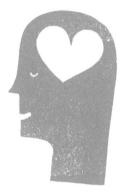

True happiness comes when
we focus less on external
things and more on our
own hearts and minds.

74

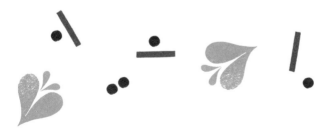

It is so easy to compare our lives to other people's, whether it's friends and family in the real world or strangers on social media. But deciding we're better or worse than someone isn't being kind to ourselves or to the people we're comparing ourselves with.

Comparison makes us unhappier. A study in the *Journal of Social and Clinical Psychology* found a link between Facebook and symptoms of depression, linked to social comparison. The study showed that whether we compare ourselves upwards (feeling like we're better than the other person), downwards (feeling like we're not as good) or neutrally, the end result is still the same – we end up feeling worse. Comparison will consume your thoughts and steal your joy – opt for happiness and kindness instead.

17

Be
PRESENT

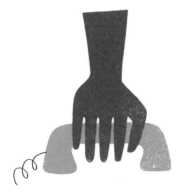

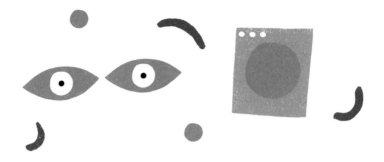

Splitting your focus
sends a clear signal to the
person you're with that
they are not worthy
of your full attention.

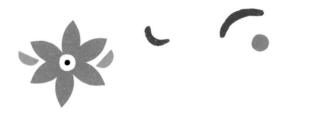

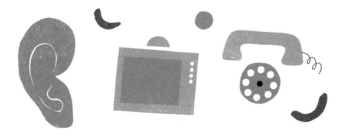

We might give people our physical presence, but how often do we give them our mental presence? Multi-tasking has become the norm for many of us – it's tempting to keep one eye on the TV, the washing or the phone while you're spending time with someone, which tells them they aren't important and not deserving of your attention.

Unlike other animals, we spend 46.9 per cent of our waking hours thinking about something other than what we're doing, according to psychologists at Harvard University. They discovered that all this mind-wandering comes at an emotional cost and typically makes us unhappy. Be mindful of how powerful your mental presence is and the effect it can have on the people in your life. Attention is a simple way to show love and one of the kindest things you can give.

#17 – BE PRESENT

18

Find a
GOOD HOME

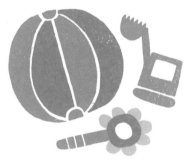

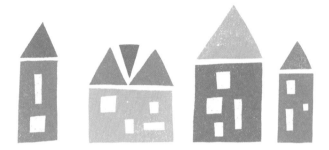

There are so many
weird and wonderful

ways to donate your

unwanted treasures.

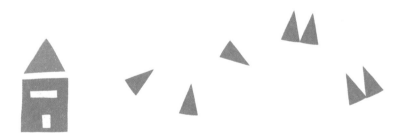

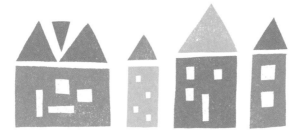

Many of us have things we don't need any more, and your unwanted goods can make someone else's life easier. Rather than just throw your possessions away, find a grateful home by donating them to someone who could really benefit.

+ Donate your old toys to a Prison Visitors' Centre to help make the experience of a visit more enjoyable for children
+ Give your old workwear to charities that help people back into the workforce
+ Consider passing on your wedding dress, bridesmaids' dresses or decorations to a charity that helps couples in need
+ Donate flowers from a funeral, wedding or event to a nursing home or local hospital
+ Gift children's books to a hospital waiting room or doctor's surgery
+ Pass on unwanted baby things to charities that help new parents
+ Donate school shoes to a local school.

Be kind to
YOURSELF

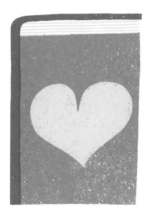

Self-love is not selfish.
Silence that inner critic
and feel good to be you.

Looking after ourselves is key to kindness, because when we feel good we emit that positive feeling to others. When we neglect ourselves, life feels like a struggle and our negative feelings influence how we interact with those around us. The author Dr Ali Binazir calculated that the probability of our being born is so low that it's practically zero. You're nothing short of a miracle! Set some time aside to celebrate. Nurture yourself by doing what you love – whether that's a warm bath, a doze in the sunshine or time listening to music – and restore your reserves not only for yourself but also for those around you.

87

Self-love can be about treating ourselves, determining to change our circumstances, deciding we need to be treated with kindness and respect, or deciding to be ourselves and not the person everyone expects us to be. These ways of being kind to ourselves make us happier, and in turn, more kind to others.

– David R. Hamilton, Ph.D.

20

FORGIVE

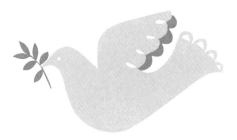

Holding a grudge against
someone or being too
hard on yourself reduces
happiness – and it's bad
for your health!

Forgive yourself and forgive other people. Forgiving someone doesn't mean condoning their behaviour, it's making a conscious decision to let go of negative feelings. You'll feel better and live longer! Chronic anger puts you into a fight-or-flight mode, causing changes in heart rate, blood pressure and immune response, according to psychiatrist Dr Karen Swartz. These changes increase the risk of developing conditions such as depression, heart disease and diabetes. Forgiveness, on the other hand, calms stress levels, leading to improved health.

91

However, the benefits depend on the nature of your forgiveness. Research by Dr Neal Krause of Michigan University suggests the outcome of forgiveness depends on how that forgiveness is given. People can either forgive unconditionally or feel the need for acts of contrition (to make amends). It is the people who forgive unconditionally that benefit from a greater sense of well-being.

21

Change a life with
GADGETS

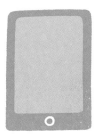

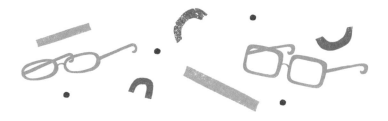

When you upgrade your technology, you can use your outdated models to help change lives and build futures.

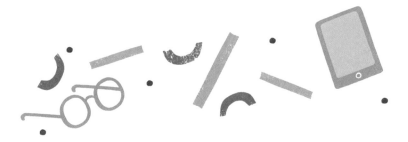

Vision therapists can use your old iPad to help people losing their sight, and schools can make use of them to help children with learning difficulties. So before you tuck your old but still usable IT away in a drawer to languish unloved, contact schools or vision therapists in your area to see if they can put it to good use.

' When we were denied funding for an iPad for my profoundly disabled son because he was too young I turned to 52 Lives, and from the bottom of my heart we can't thank them enough. The most beautiful feeling swept over me because it was confirmation that good people are out there and want to help someone they have never met. Harrison got his iPad and it is helping to improve his vision, and we will be able to use the communication apps in the future to help him and us understand each other better. No one will ever know how grateful we are. '

– *Hayley, who has seen first-hand the difference technology can make for someone in need*

22

Give

ENCOURAGEMENT

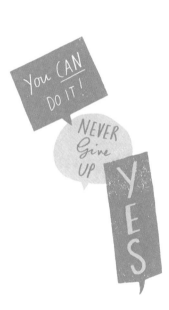

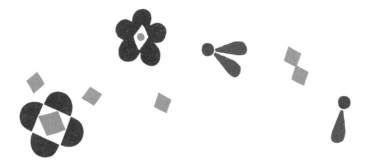

Your words can nourish people's ideas and help them become something amazing.

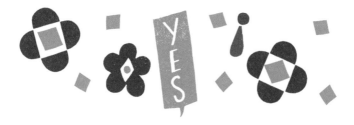

If we look for it, there is always fault to be found, but positivity is the best way to help someone succeed. Encouragement can inspire people to dream, to believe in themselves and to take action towards their goals. Be kind – choose to be an encourager rather than a critic and you will unleash more creativity, resourcefulness and happiness than you could imagine.

'Focusing on what someone needs to do to "fix" themselves will close them down to new possibilities or ideas. Whereas positivity and encouragement activates parts of the limbic system that allow you to be more open and positive, as well as the visual cortex, which enables imagination.'

– Richard Boyatzis, Ph.D., professor and author of Primal Leadership

23

Hug with
HEART

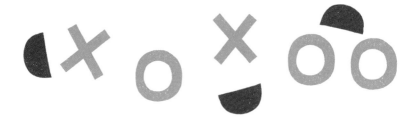

When you hug someone,
make it count. Hug
with love – and often.

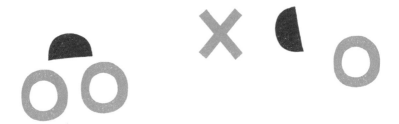

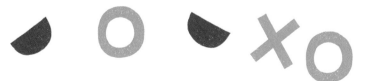

I call them 'hugs with hearts' – all-in, chests together, arms wrapped tightly all the way around. They are what my children give me for my birthday! But try not to save your hugs with heart for special occasions. With one powerful embrace, you can help someone you care about feel amazing, and it has the added benefit of simultaneously helping you to feel good.

🔍 Hugging is a simple way to keep oxytocin flowing. Scientist and author Dr Paul Zak (otherwise known as 'Dr Love') says this interpersonal touch raises oxytocin, reduces cardiovascular stress and improves the immune system. So rather than a half-hearted hug or a handshake, hug with heart – Dr Zak prescribes eight a day. You really can hug someone better.

Make special occasions special

FOR EVERYONE

24

On celebration days,
spread kindness to those
who may be struggling.

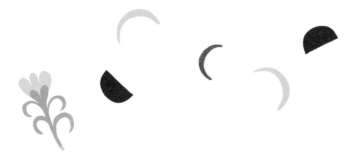

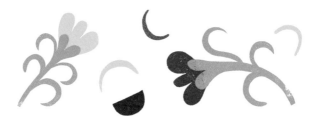

For people who have lost someone, special days such as birthdays, Mother's Day or Father's Day can serve as reminders that the person they loved is no longer around. Letting them know you're thinking of them can ease their pain, even a little. For people who have no one, think about how you can help them feel included – give a gift to a homeless person, visit an elderly person who's on their own ... whatever you can do to make special days special for everyone.

❝ Miriam's ninth birthday was approaching and it was going to be the first since her little brother, Abyan, had passed away. Miriam was upset he wouldn't be by her side. Strangers came forward to throw a surprise party and create a memorial garden so she could have happy place think about Abyan. She had the most amazing birthday. ❞

— *Laila (Miriam's mum). 52 Lives supporters sent cards and gifts, threw a surprise party for this little girl after she lost her brother*

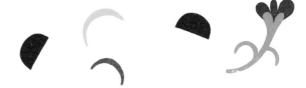

25

Pay
FOR TWO

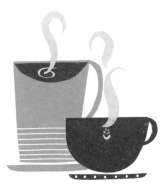

If you can afford a little bit
extra, consider buying two
things instead of one as
you go about your day.

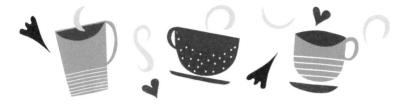

Some cafés run a 'suspended coffee' scheme to help spread kindness, where you can buy food or drinks for people in need to reclaim later. And for those cafés or outlets that don't already do this, asking whether you can may prompt them to start – pay for someone's coffee, buy an extra sandwich, or pay for two field trips at school in case a family can't afford it.

One morning, just before Christmas in 2012, a Tim Hortons' coffee shop in Canada became famous for a chain of kindness that spontaneously occurred at its drive-through window. A customer paid for her order and also paid the bill for the stranger in the car behind. That customer then decided to do the same for the car behind them ... this continued for the next 226 customers, in a three-hour kindness spree. Kindness inspires kindness!

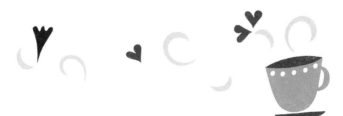

26

Take the
INITIATIVE

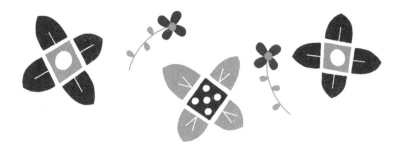

People who need help can
be shy about asking for it –
maybe they think the world
is against them or they
don't want to be a burden.

114

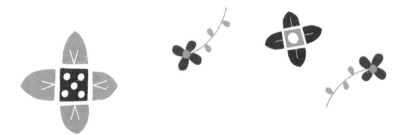

*If you think someone could do with some help, take the
initiative. Offer to carry a pram up the stairs, take a meal
to someone undergoing chemo, carry someone's tray
if they have their hands full … It doesn't matter if they
decline. A kind offer is never wasted.*

'Immediately after Fiona died was a stressful time. I had
to quit my job, work out how to make ends meet and,
most importantly, support my daughters. When we were
offered help, my initial response was to say thanks but
no thanks. But as the weeks went on, things got harder,
so I put my pride aside. People made meals and dropped
them around. The idea that someone would take time out
of their life to make ours a little easier was really special.'

— *Stewart was helped by staff from a local business (Crick
Auto Group) after his wife suddenly passed away. The
Crick team helps change one life a month, as part of
a partnership with 52 Lives*

27

Be happy for people's
HAPPINESS

Happiness is not finite, and someone else's good fortune doesn't take away your own potential for happiness.

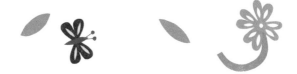

When something good happens to someone you know, celebrate their success. Sometimes when another person is happy about something or their lives change in a positive way, feelings of envy can creep in and taint our behaviour. Try to choose happiness over envy and delight in their good fortune. Their win is not your loss – it's an opportunity for the selfless celebration of someone else's joy. If you ever find it hard to feel happy for someone, see it as a chance to be kind to yourself and to them. Ask yourself:

+ What could I do to be kind to this person?
+ What do I have to be grateful for? (Gratitude is a powerful antidote to envy)
+ Am I being bigger than envy? (Banish small-mindedness)
+ Is there anything I could do in my own life to bring me more happiness?
+ Does this person's happiness diminish mine?
+ Was I content before I heard about this?
+ Does this really matter? (Having perspective always helps).

#27 – BE HAPPY FOR PEOPLE'S HAPPINESS

28

Give people the benefit
OF THE DOUBT

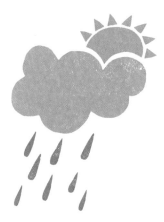

None of us know what is
going on in someone's life.
122   If someone is behaving
in a way you don't like,
try to be understanding.

The person that sped past you might be in the middle of a crisis, the person who was abrupt might have had some bad news, and the child misbehaving might be having a tough time at home. Thinking the worst of people will bring you down and reduce your capacity for kindness. Choose to think the best of everyone instead.

❝ One day, I asked my students to fill in the blank in this sentence: "I wish my teacher knew _____." These were some of the responses:
+ "Sometimes my homework is not signed because my mum is not around a lot."
+ "My family lives in a shelter."
+ "My dad died this year and I feel more alone than ever before." ❞

— *Kyle Schwartz is the author of* I Wish My Teacher Knew. *52 Lives supporters bought warm coats and jackets for the children in her class*

29

Thank the
UNAPPRECIATED

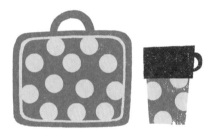

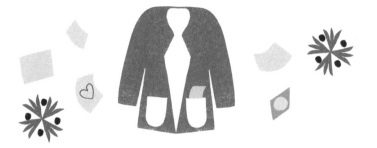

Show the people in your
life that you appreciate
what they do, whether they
are your main cast or your
background crew.

There are so many people that make up the fabric of lives, and sometimes we forget they are even there. But feeling valued can have a profound effect on our self-worth by adding meaning to our lives. It also helps us feel more confident, happier and motivated. So take a few moments to thank those who are often unappreciated …

+ Leave a Post-it note in your child's lunchbox
+ Hide a letter in your partner's pocket
+ Tape a thank you to your front door for your postman
+ Say thank you to your bus driver
+ Write a thank you note to your child's teacher and tuck it into their homework
+ Thank the person serving you during busy periods when others might be complaining
+ Thank the behind-the-scenes staff at your workplace or school, who keep it clean or running smoothly.

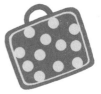

#29 – THANK THE UNAPPRECIATED

30

Embrace
CURIOSITY

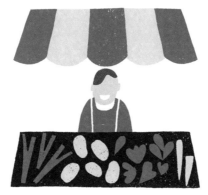

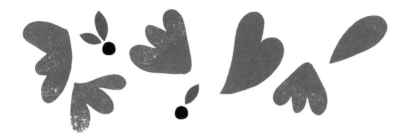

Taking an interest in others may broaden your mind and lead to new discoveries, which in itself can cause a hit of feel-good brain chemicals!

When you talk to people, how often do you ask questions?
Are you usually in 'transmit' mode or do you encourage
others to talk? Whether you're surrounded by strangers,
or with your loved ones, try to learn about people. Find
out what they do, things they've done or what they think.
Being curious about those around us brings a whole range
of benefits. It combats people's loneliness, creates a sense
of community and helps us feel we are worth something.
Setting yourself a challenge to learn more about those
around you will open you up to new experiences, learning
new things, and it can provide a natural boost to your
dopamine levels.

🔎 Dopamine is one of the chemicals responsible for
transmitting signals in between the nerve cells (neurons)
of the brain, explains Dr Phil Newton from Swansea
University. But it's best-known for being our brain's
'pleasure centre', providing positive feelings to motivate
us to do, or continue doing, certain things.

31

Laugh
ABOUT IT!

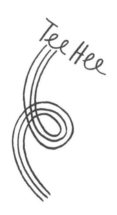

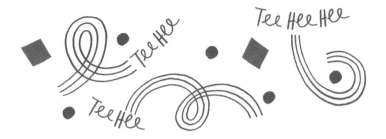

Taking things (even serious
things) a bit less seriously
can be kinder on everyone.

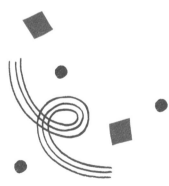

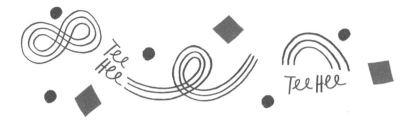

Sometimes life can feel heavy – we all have worries that occupy our minds and they can consume us if we let them. Every now and then, remind yourself not to take life too seriously and help those around you have fun. Lighten the mood, laugh about things, enjoy the journey and try not to hold on to those worrying thoughts for too long. It can brighten a loved one's dark times, even for just a few moments, and it can make life a lot less stressful for you too.

' When I was recovering from cancer, I would have loved to have more fun experiences – my friends were a great support, but it was mostly sitting around chatting and everyone was so serious with me all the time. I wanted to laugh and be normal and feel alive. '

– A 52 Lives supporter who survived cancer

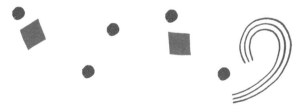

#31 – LAUGH ABOUT IT!

32

Give away a
MINUTE

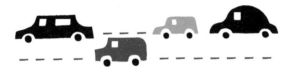

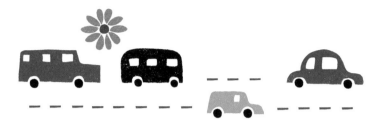

By having patience and being courteous to people, for even one minute a day, you can make a positive difference.

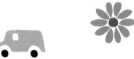

Could you give away one minute of your day to create a kinder world? Try to leave home a minute earlier than usual so you have time to be more thoughtful, let someone ahead of you in a queue and let other cars in when you're driving. Would you rather be the angry person honking their horn or the calm soul waving someone through?

139

'Not only does patience benefit others but it is also good for you! Research shows that of the different types of patience people may possess (such as patience with life hardships, daily hassles, or people), patience with other people is most predictive of personal well-being. Moreover, incorporating intentional practices into daily life to increase patience can increase positive emotions and decrease depressive symptoms. Some people think that cultivating patience will make them timid or a "doormat", but this is not what we find in our research. Patience actually facilitates goal achievement across time and is independent from assertiveness.'

— *Sarah A. Schnitker, Ph.D., Thrive Centre for Human Development*

33

Give
WISHES

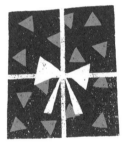

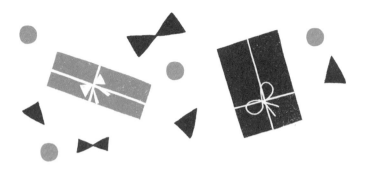

Next time you're celebrating
a special occasion, such as
a birthday or wedding, ask
your friends to donate money
to your favourite charity
instead of buying gifts.

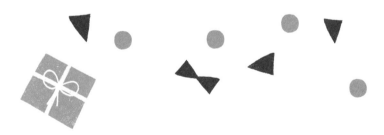

At 52 Lives, we often create wish lists for the people
we help and fill them with all the things they need. Kind
strangers then buy the gifts. It's a practical and selfless
way of spreading kindness. As well as asking friends to
donate to a charity, you could set up an Amazon wish list
for someone in need of help and ask your friends to fulfil it.

' I really don't want or use a lot of things, and my house
needs de-cluttering rather than more things added to
it. I know people like to spoil their friends and family,
so asking them not to buy presents on special occasions
seems ungrateful. Instead, I suggest they send any money
they would have spent on my gift to a good cause, and let
me know what they have done. It's lovely to think about
my "presents" giving help to people who really need it. '

— A 52 Lives supporter

#33 – GIVE WISHES

34

Beware of busyness leading
TO UNKINDNESS

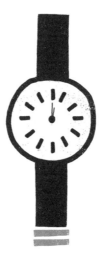

When we have too
much to do, it leaves
little room for us to think
about other people.

There will always be things in life that try to demand our immediate attention – deadlines, missed calls or a full inbox. But busyness is the death of kindness; we have little time for anything or anyone else. Prioritise your personal well-being and try to focus your energy on what's important, rather than what seems urgent. It will free up your time and your mind to spend on the things that matter to you, with the people you love. The average family spends just over half an hour a day together 'undistracted' – time where they feel they actually bond together and catch up without anything else getting in the way, according to research commissioned by Highland Spring.

Author and founder of *Becoming Minimalist*, Joshua Becker, suggests we find freedom in saying 'no' to less important commitments in order to open up our lives to pursue the most important. Sometimes having less, doing less and expecting less can help us gain more of the things we actually need.

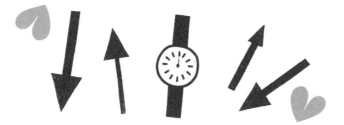

35

Create beautiful
SPACES

Rather than seeing rubbish
as a blight on the landscape,
see it as an opportunity to
be kind to the community.

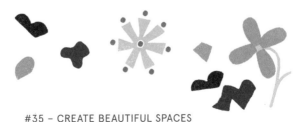

*Instead of feeling cross about how horrible it looks, aim
to pick up a few pieces of rubbish you spot each day. We
tend to care for our environment more when it is already
in a good state, so your small act may inspire others to
do the same.*

As well as creating beautiful spaces, picking up rubbish
could also help keep your neighbourhood safe. A survey
by Keep Britain Tidy showed places that have the lowest
levels of litter, fly-posting and graffiti are also those least
at risk from crime. This relates to what's known as the
'broken windows theory', which says that maintaining
urban environments to prevent small crimes helps to
create an atmosphere of order and lawfulness, which
then prevents more serious crimes.

#35 – CREATE BEAUTIFUL SPACES

36

Be
HONEST

Forget about airbrushing
your life and choose to
be authentic instead.

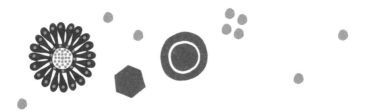

It's common to try to present ourselves in the best possible light. Sometimes we put on a glossy front and don't say how we are really feeling. Being honest about our thoughts, our lives and our feelings is a form of kindness. It gives other people the freedom to be honest as well, by creating a safe and authentic space where we can say how we really feel and be who we truly are. It makes for real conversations and improves the well-being of everyone around us. It is also one of the most liberating things you can do for yourself – so shake off the shackles of perfection and be your real self.

Being dishonest is tied in with our self-esteem. Research by psychologist Robert Feldman found that as soon as people feel that their self-esteem is threatened, they immediately begin to lie at higher levels. Men lie the same amount as women, but they tend to lie to make themselves look better, while women are more likely to lie to make the other person feel better.

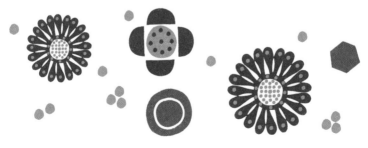

#36 – BE HONEST

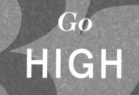

37

Go
HIGH

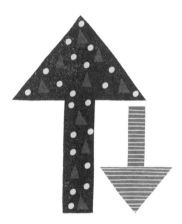

Rise above toxicity and choose positivity. It's good for the soul and gives us a natural high.

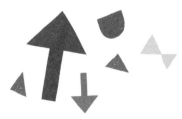

Former First Lady Michelle Obama famously said, 'When they go low, we go high.' Sometimes we find ourselves in toxic environments – whether it be with people who are overly negative, or involved in conversations that are nasty, gossipy or unhelpful. It can be tempting to go along with things to be agreeable or to avoid conflict, but next time you're in that situation, try to be the person that goes 'high'. Stooping to the level of those around you will have a negative effect on your mind and body, and add more toxicity to the world. Choosing to 'go high' will boost your feel-good brain chemicals and you might even convert a few negative people along the way.

Kindness changes our brain chemistry. It boosts levels of dopamine and serotonin, which are chemical messengers involved with positive emotions. It also produces oxytocin, the 'bonding hormone'. It even produces endorphins, the brain's natural versions of morphine and heroin. Kindness really does give us a totally legal high.

— *David R. Hamilton, Ph.D., from* The Five Side Effects of Kindness

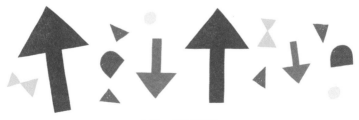

#37 – GO HIGH

38

Be kind in
A CRISIS

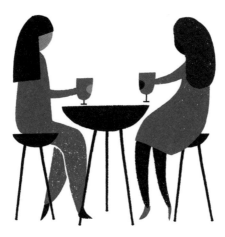

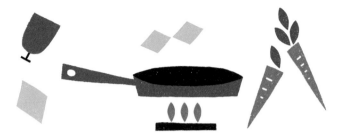

We aren't always sure of the
best way to help, or we are

afraid of saying or doing the
wrong thing. But your kindness
can make a big difference.

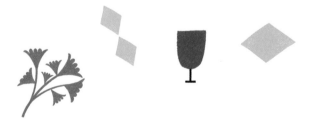

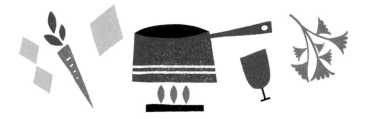

When someone goes through a big life event – whether having a baby, being diagnosed with a serious illness or getting a divorce – think about ways you can help. Try not to worry about doing the 'right' or 'wrong' thing – the gesture itself is less important than the love and thoughtfulness that comes with it. But here are some ideas to help get you started …

+ Follow up – support often floods in for someone in the short term, but make sure you check in with people a few weeks or months on
+ Cook a healthy meal and drop it over
+ Offer to pick up groceries
+ Do their school run or babysit
+ Clean their house
+ Deliver some fun – lighten the mood, laugh with them or take them out in the world
+ Demonstrate your offer to help is genuine by asking specifically what you can help with, or make suggestions. Sometimes this allows people to be more honest.

39

Give
SILENCE

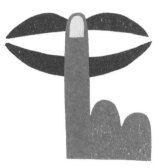

Your silence is kindness.
It's where ideas flourish,
real human connection
happens, and genuine
friendships are forged.

166

When we ask someone how they are, sometimes we're just waiting for our turn to speak. And so we interrupt with a question, an observation or to talk about ourselves. We might think we're helping people by giving them the answers, or by hurrying the conversation along, but what we are doing is cutting off their thoughts and ideas, and making the relationship a more superficial one. When someone is allowed to speak, it uncovers truths and emotions that would otherwise be left unsaid. This week, ask someone how they are then give them a whole minute of airtime, without saying a word.

Silence gets you out of the way and creates a space others will fill in with themselves. For this to happen, it might require us to train ourselves to be silent – to consciously make ourselves wait far beyond the point that feels comfortable.

— *Dr Alex Lickerman, author of* The Undefeated Mind

#39 – GIVE SILENCE

40

Let
KINDNESS IN

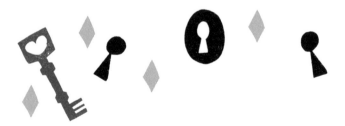

Accepting help might seem weak, but there is so much strength in vulnerability.

We might feel too proud, too guilty or just uncomfortable accepting kindness, but be good to yourself – admit when you need some help and try to believe that you are worthy of kindness. It will help both you and the person offering you help – allow them to feel good about helping you.

'Sometimes the hardest thing is to ask for help. We try not to ask because we don't want to disturb people or we just feel like this is our battle ... this is our life and we don't want people to be obliged to help. It's hard even to ask our friends for help, let alone people we don't know. So when people who are strangers helped us with the things we need – there are just no words for how that felt. You think this world is a mad place, but it isn't. There's so many good people out there. The original human is kind.'

— *Onessa's severely ill son, Elijah, was helped by 52 Lives supporters. They gave Elijah's bedroom a makeover, bought some essential items for him, and sent his parents away for a weekend break*

41

Be GRATEFUL

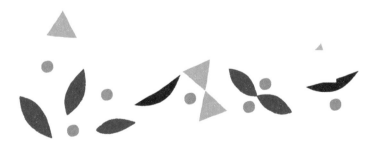

Being grateful helps us feel happier, less envious, less attached to material things and much more open to being kind to those around us.

It's impossible to feel grateful and angry at the same time, so start and end your day thinking about all the things you have to be thankful for. There is always something … having someone who cares about you, fresh air in your lungs, food, shelter, or the capacity to love. Showing gratitude for even the littlest things that make up our day – a good cup of coffee, a few minutes of extra sleep or a beautiful flower in the garden – can have a positive effect on our well-being and increase our capacity for kindness.

175

People who are grateful tend to be happier than those who are not. A study compared people keeping a list of their blessings with people listing their hassles and found that the blessings group were 25 per cent happier than the hassles group, feeling more joyful, enthusiastic, strong and attentive.

— *David R Hamilton, Ph.D., from* Why Kindness is Good For You

42

Have
PERSPECTIVE

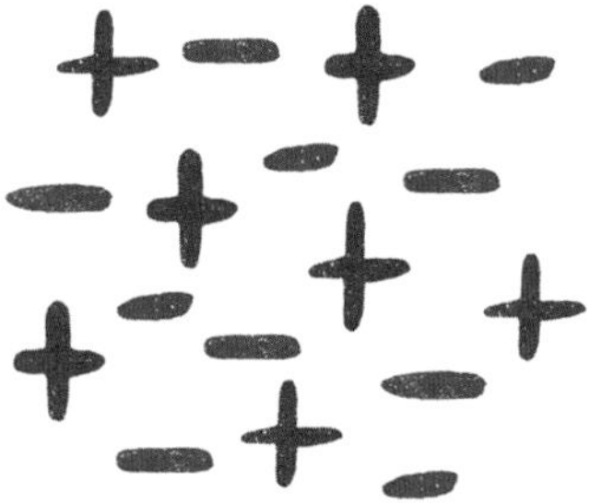

When you're worried, upset
or angry about something,
your negative emotions can
rub off on those around you.

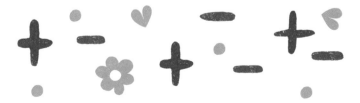

So next time you're feeling particularly anxious or annoyed, step back and ask yourself if what you're upset about really matters. When we zoom out and look at the bigger picture, there are very few things worth worrying about. Your calm approach will also help create a more kind, loving environment for those around you. Just as the effect of smiles and positive emotions can be passed on from those around us, negative emotions can also be 'caught' – especially from those closest to us.

179

Researchers in Japan found that emotional contagion was significantly stronger among friends and family than acquaintances, suggesting the degree of intimacy we have with someone influences how susceptible we are to picking up their emotions.

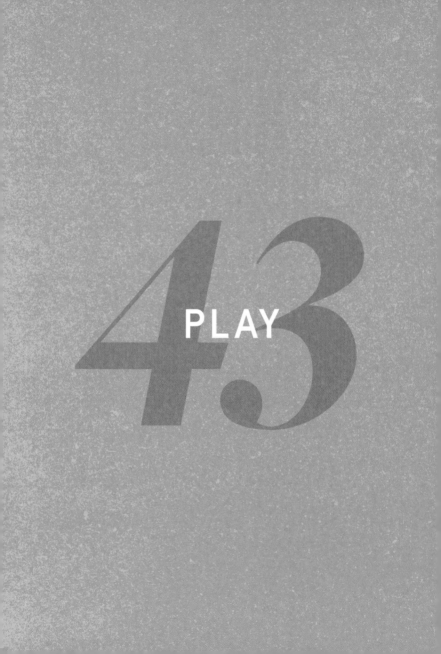

PLAY 43

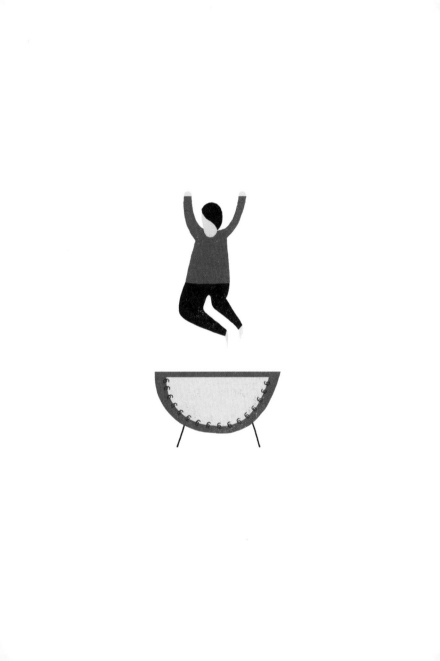

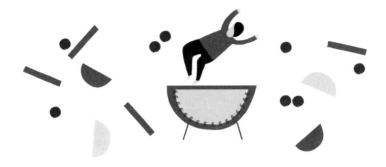

When we play, it distracts

our minds from everyday

life and allows us to re-set.

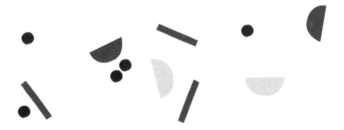

Whether it's making a game out of your daily tasks, setting yourself small challenges, or physically sitting down to play a game, try to introduce some playtime into your life.

Playing games is a great antidote to stress and helps us to connect and bond with those around us. And when we feel more relaxed and connected, we are more likely to show kindness. According to author and gaming guru Jane McGonigal, playing produces powerful emotions and social relationships that can change our lives and the lives of those around us. Her research found that it provokes our most powerful positive emotions (curiosity, optimism and pride) and strengthens relationships with friends and family.

— *Jane McGonigal is the author of* SuperBetter *and* Reality is Broken. *Jane was bedridden and suicidal following a severe concussion and used games to heal herself*

44

Be aware of your
THOUGHTS

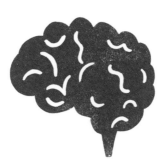

Being aware of where
your feelings are coming
from will help you avoid
blaming those around you,
and take responsibility
for your own feelings.

It's common to blame others for how we are feeling, in the process damaging relationships and creating hostility. Your boss gave you too much work, so you feel stressed; your friend was rude, so you feel upset; or, more positively, your partner was kind, so you feel happy. But that's not how humans work: our feelings can only come from our thoughts about a situation – not from the situation itself.

Both neuroscience and physics are now pointing to the fact that the human experience is created from the inside out. This reveals a huge misunderstanding. Our realities are not being passively recorded by the brain, but are actively constructed by it in every moment. Admittedly our thoughts can portray the illusion that our experience is coming from something outside of ourselves, but it is all coming from within. Realising that gives us more psychological freedom, resourcefulness and compassion.

— *Piers Thurston is a mindset and state-of-mind trainer at organisational change consultancy, Making Change Work*

#44 – BE AWARE OF YOUR THOUGHTS

VOLUNTEER

45

Time can be a difficult
thing for us to give, which
is why it's such a generous
way of being kind.

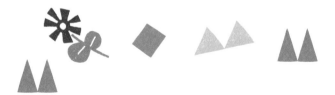

Devoting some of your time to others will bring more benefits than you might expect. Not only will you be helping people, but you will also be helping yourself. Volunteering has been shown to combat depression and boost happiness in those who give their time.

' I've struggled with my mental health and I've realised that the smallest acts of kindness can mean the world. When 52 Lives helped me I was so grateful because to me, it wasn't just material donations, it was people believing in me. That's why I started The Comfort Project. I want people who are struggling with mental illness to feel worthy of love, dignity and respect. By helping others I am helping myself. I still struggle with my mental health, but even helping one other person can make a world of difference. '

— Emmeline was helped by 52 Lives and went on to launch her own project, providing essential items to people in mental-health units

46

Save a
LIFE

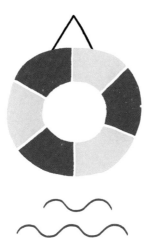

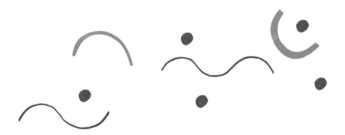

With just the things in
your body, you can save
a life. It doesn't get much
kinder than that!

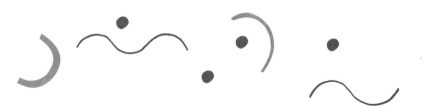

And whether it's life-saving organs, or life-changing hair, there are so many different things from your own body that you can donate to make someone else's life better. For example, your hair could make a wig for a child with cancer, your umbilical cord blood could prevent an amputation, your bone marrow could provide life-saving treatment, and your stem cells could help someone beat leukaemia. Go online or talk to your doctor to find out what you can do to help.

‘ I was nervous and then when I got on to the bed I was really nervous. But it was fine. It was just a little pinch. I feel happy and helpful that I could do it for her. I like helping people. ’

— *Five-year-old Oliver donated bone marrow and stem cells to save his sister's life*

47

Heal with
KINDNESS

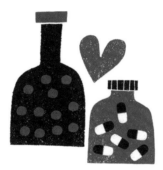

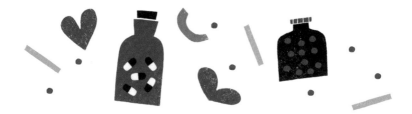

Sometimes we might feel
there is nothing we can
do to help someone who's
ill, but showing kindness
is a proven way of helping
people to recover.

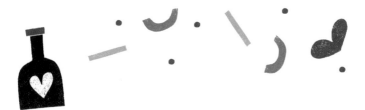

Your kindness can act as a medicine. Research has revealed that people shown kindness experience faster healing of wounds, less pain and anxiety, reduced blood pressure and shorter hospital stays. Best of all, kindness has healing properties for both the giver and the receiver, so it will benefit you too.

' When I was seven, I was diagnosed with stage 4 cancer in my kidney. It had spread to my veins and my lungs, and I was so lucky to survive. Years later, I met the doctor who saved my life, and thanked him for what he did for me. I'll never forget what he said – "I didn't save your life, your parents did." Never underestimate the effect that love and kindness can have on people who are ill. I wouldn't be here now without it. '

– *Greig Trout, double cancer survivor and founder of 101 Things to Do When You Survive*

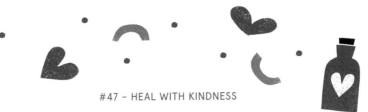

#47 – HEAL WITH KINDNESS

48

Be
ACCEPTING

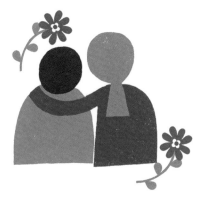

Accepting people as they are, rather than trying to change them, will help them become the best possible versions of themselves.

*Treat people in your life with love, understanding and
acceptance and watch them flourish. Feeling accepted
and supported boosts our self-worth, which can unlock
potential and help us thrive. So try not to judge – sometimes
the kindest thing to do is nothing, apart from to love.
Here are seven steps to help you become more accepting …*

203

+ Listen with an open mind
+ Be aware your beliefs may be different to those of
  others. That doesn't mean they're wrong
+ Remember that people act with good intentions – they
  think what they're doing is the best way forward, even
  if you disagree
+ If what you're thinking isn't either helpful or kind,
  perhaps stay quiet
+ Always focus on the good – in the situation and in
  the person
+ Be aware that the traits we dislike in someone else are often
  the traits we fear we ourselves have. We are all fallible
+ Show love and compassion. It can only help – it will
  never make things worse.

49

Give without
EXPECTATION

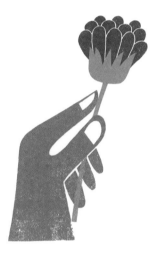

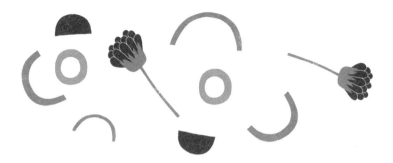

Showing kindness without expecting anything in return is kindness in its purest form.

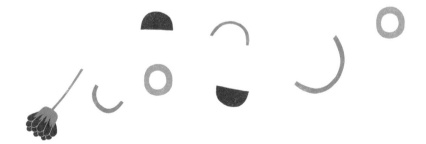

Experiencing the joy of giving is your reward, and even if no one ever knows what you have done, or the person you help doesn't thank you, you will know that you made a difference in someone's life. That really is all that matters.

' There is something inside of me that doesn't feel right if I don't help when I know I can. If we are in a position to ease someone else's suffering, I feel we should. Loneliness is at the heart of so much pain in life. Feeling alone, struggling day-to-day thinking nobody cares about you is mentally exhausting. We should all be helping each other to heal in these times of great need. Kindness and compassion is liberating, and friendship, love and understanding helps us all carry on in this crazy little thing called life. '

– *A 52 Lives supporter who donated a car anonymously to a single mum and her son, who both had cancer*

50

Build an
ARMY

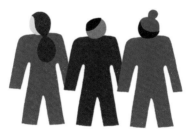

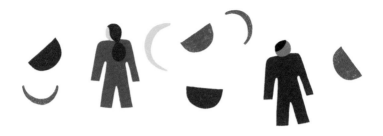

When an army of kind
people comes together
to do good, the
possibilities are limitless.

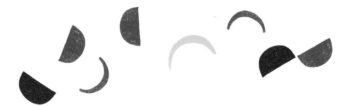

As an individual, helping someone can sometimes feel overwhelming. So if you know someone in need of help, but can't do it on your own, spread the word among family and friends – when everyone helps a little bit, giving becomes a whole lot easier.

' I've seen how isolating and demanding having a poorly sibling can be. I wanted to do something to show siblings how super they are but I realised I couldn't do it alone. I thought with a little bit of kindness from a lot of people, I could make a big difference, so I launched "Sponsor a Sibling." With the help of many strangers, we have formed an army. '

– Laura, founder of Sponsor a Sibling. Laura's son, Harry, has Batten disease, and 52 Lives supporters bought him a hoist. Laura then went on to launch her charity, which sends gifts to siblings of poorly children

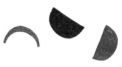

51

Make Kindness
A THING

Let's create a world where people are idolised for who they are – not for what they have, how pretty they are or what they do for a living.

214

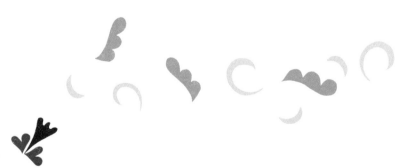

Kindness is a powerful force for change and, I believe, the most important quality a person can have. We can all help to make sure it is valued as such, not treated as an optional extra. Let's praise people for their kindness, admire them for their actions and help make kindness the thing to be most proud of.

When we asked one of the children who took part in the 52 Lives School Kindness Project what they wanted to be when they were older, this is what they said: 'I want to be kind when I grow up. And smiley. Smiley and kind.' 52 Lives visits a different school each week to run Kindness workshops that empower children and encourage them to value kindness.

#51 – MAKE KINDNESS A THING

52

Give a copy of
THIS BOOK

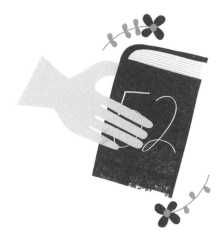

To help spread the word,
give a copy of this book to

218 someone or leave one where

someone can find it. Release

kindness into the world!

You read all the way to the end – thank you! I hope this book has filled you with ideas of little ways you can make a significant difference, both to yourself and the people around you, simply by being kind.

It is the little choices we make every day that determine the kind of world we live in, so always choose kindness. When we're kind to one person, it might actually be affecting around 16 people, believes Dr David Hamilton. Hamilton bases this figure on research which shows that our behaviour has a three-stage knock-on, or 'ripple', effect – so when we help one person, that person then helps other people, who in turn help others. He calls this the '3-Degree Ripple Rule'. Choosing kindness on a daily basis will spark a change in yourself, your family, your community ... and eventually the world!

#52 – GIVE A COPY OF THIS BOOK

Appendix & useful websites

52 Lives
www.52-lives.org
www.facebook.com/52lives
www.twitter.com/52lives
www.instagram.com/52.lives

#02 Hamilton, David R. *The Five Side Effects of Kindness*
(Hay House, 2017)

#03 Find your local food bank: www.trusselltrust.org (UK),
www.feedingamerica.org (US), www.foodbank.org.au (Australia)

#04 Do Something for Nothing: www.dosomethingfornothing.net

#05 Hamilton, David R.: www.drdavidhamilton.com

#06 Dscout 'Mobile Touches Study', June 2016: www.dscout.com
Teo, A. R., Choi, H., Valenstein, M. (2013), 'Social Relationships and
Depression: Ten-Year Follow-Up from a Nationally Representative
Study'. *PLoS ONE* 8(4): e62396. www.doi.org/10.1371/journal.
pone.0062396

#09 Lyubomirsky, S. *The How of Happiness* (Piatkus, 2010)

#11 Hamilton, David R. *The Five Side Effects of Kindness*
(Hay House, 2017)
Stout, C., Morrow, J., Brandt, E., Wolf, S. (1964), 'Unusually Low Incidence
of Death From Myocardial Infarction: Study of an Italian American
Community in Pennsylvania' (*Journal of the American Medical
Association*, 188, 845–849).

#12 Lewicki, R. J., Lount, R. B., Polin, B. (May 2016), 'An Exploration
of the Structure of Effective Apologies', *Negotiation and Conflict
Management Research*

#15 The Happy News: www.thehappynewspaper.com

#16 Steers, M.-L., Wickham, R., Acitelli, L. (2014), 'Seeing Everyone
Else's Highlight Reels: How Facebook Usage is Linked to Depressive
Symptoms', *Journal of Social and Clinical Psychology*, 33 (8), 701–731

#17 Gilbert, Killingsworth (2010), Harvard University, 'A Wandering Mind Is an
Unhappy Mind', *Science*, 330 (6006), 932

#18 Donating workwear: Suited and Booted (UK) www.suitedbootedcentre.
org.uk Dress for Success (global) www.dressforsuccess.org
Donating wedding goods: The Wedding Wishing Well Foundation
(UK) www.weddingwishingwell.org.uk; Gift of a Wedding (UK)
www.giftofawedding.org; Brides for a Cause (US)
www.bridesforacause.com
Donating baby goods: Baby Bank Network (UK):
www.babybanknetwork.com; Baby2Baby (US): www.baby2baby.org;
Dandelion Support Network (Australia): www.dandelionsupport.org.au

#19 Hamilton, David R.: www.drdavidhamilton.com
Binazir, Dr Ali: www.blogs.harvard.edu/abinazir/2011/06/15/
what-are-chances-you-would-be-born

#20 Dr Karen Swartz, Director of the Mood Disorders Adult Consultation
Clinic at The Johns Hopkins Hospital in 'Forgiveness: Your Health
Depends on It', www.hopkinsmedicine.org
Neal Krause, Marshall H. Becker Collegiate Professor
Emeritus, Department of Health Behavior and Health
Education, School of Public Health, University of Michigan
Krause, N. (2016), 'Compassion, Acts of Contrition, and Forgiveness in
Middle and Late Life', *Pastoral Psychology*, 65(1), 127–141

#22 Richard Boyatzis, Professor, Departments of Organizational
Behavior, Psychology, and Cognitive Science, Case Western
Reserve University.

#23 Zak, Paul. *The Morale Molecule* (Corgi, 2013), www.pauljzak.com

#26 Cricks 12 Lives: www.cricks12lives.com.au

#28 Schwartz, Kyle. *I Wish My Teacher Knew* (Da Capo Lifelong Books,
2016). www.iwishmyteacherknewbook.com

#30 Dr Phil Newton is Director of Learning and Teaching at Swansea
University Medical School. www.psychologytoday.com/
blog/mouse-man/200904/what-is-dopamine

#32 Thomas, R. M., Schnitker, S. A. (in press). 'Modeling the
Effects of Within-Person Characteristic and Goal-Level Attributes
on Personal Project Pursuit Over Time', *Journal of Research in
Personality*. Advance online publication. doi:10.1016/j.jrp.2016.06.012
Schnitker, S. A., (2012), 'An examination of patience and well-being',
Journal of Positive Psychology, 7, 263–280. doi:10.1080/17439760.
2012.697185

#34 Highland Spring study into family time: www.highlandspringgroup.com/
press-and-media/group-news/article/34-minutes-the-amount-of-
time-the-average-family-gets-to-spend-together-each-day/

Becker, Joshua. *A Helpful Guide to Becoming Unbusy,*
www.becomingminimalist.com/un-busy/

#35 Keep Britain Tidy (2015): 'How Clean is England?' The Local
Environmental Quality Survey of England and 2014/15,
commissioned by Defra

#36 Feldman, R. S., Forrest, J. A., Happ, B. R. (2002), 'Self-presentation
and verbal deception: Do self-presenters lie more?'
Basic and Applied Social Psychology, 24, 163-170

#37 Hamilton, David R. *The Five Side Effects of Kindness*
(Hay House, 2017)

#41 Hamilton, David R. *Why Kindness Is Good for You*
(Hay House, 2010)
Emmons, Robert A., McCullough, Michael E. (Feb 2003), 'Counting
blessings versus burdens: An experimental investigation of gratitude
and subjective well-being in daily life.' *Journal of Personality and
Social Psychology*, 84(2), 377-389

#42 Kimura, M., Daibo, I., Yogo M. (2008), 'The Study of Emotional
Contagion From the Perspective of Interpersonal Relationships',
Social Behavior and Personality, An International Journal, 36(1), 27–42

#43 McGonigal, J. *Reality Is Broken: Why Games Make Us Better and How
They Can Change the World* (Vintage, 2012)

#44 Making Change Work: www.makingchangework.co.uk

#45 The Comfort Project: www.facebook.com/thecomfortprojectuk

#47 Stanford University's Center for Compassion and Altruism Research
and Education (CCARE)
Dignity Health (2014), The Healing Power of Kindness.
www.dignityhealth.org
101 Things To Do When You Survive: www.whenyousurvive.com

#50 Sponsor a Sibling: www.sponsorasibling.co.uk

#51 52 Lives School Kindness Project: www.52-lives.org/schools

#52 Hamilton, David R. *The Five Side Effects of Kindness*
(Hay House, 2017)
Fowler, J. H., Christakis, N. A. (2010). 'Cooperative behavior cascades
in human social networks'. *Proceedings of the National Academy of
Sciences of the United States of America*, 107(12), 5334–5338.
www.doi.org/10.1073/pnas.0913149107

Acknowledgements

So many people and organisations have been involved in making 52 Lives what it is today, and in bringing this book to life.

+ First and foremost, the incredible 52 Lives supporters who help change lives every single week, and never seem to tire of me asking for help! Without you, 52 Lives simply wouldn't exist.

+ Our corporate sponsor, GalaBingo.com. The team at Gala raises funds for 52 Lives each week. Thanks to their support, 100 per cent of what people give goes directly to the people we help. Gala's support keeps the charity running and enables us to do what we do. Thank you so much.

+ The lovely team at Clarins for having such faith in me. The prize money I received from the Clarins Woman of the Year Award allowed us to launch the School Kindness Project, reaching the hearts and minds of tens of thousands of children.

+ My literary agent, Jen Christie from Graham Maw Christie, who has been an incredible source of ideas, inspiration and advice. Jen, without you I'm not sure this book would exist.

+ Dr David Hamilton, for his wisdom, his science and his patience with my many, many questions.

+ Carolyn Thorne and the team at HarperCollins for their amazing enthusiasm, for embracing kindness and for turning my words into such a beautiful book.

+ Lucy Sykes-Thompson for her superb design and Debbie Powell for her beautiful illustrations.

+ My trustees, Piers, Barry and Richard, for their guidance, huge ambition and faith in my vision (or lack thereof at times!) for 52 Lives.

+ My lovely friend and colleague, Lou, who organises pretty much everything. Your colour-coded spreadsheets are a thing of beauty and I don't know what I'd do without you.

+ Dan from Einstein Tax, Cath from Candid Communications
and Adele from Magrath, for donating their time and advice to
52 Lives.

+ Orchard Wealth Management and Crick Auto Group for partnering
with us to help change people's lives every month.

+ Piers, the mindset guru, for helping me understand how human
beings work.

+ My mum and dad, for bringing out the kindness in all four of us by
giving us nothing but love. It would have been impossible to be
brought up by you and NOT be kind. And to John, Julie and Jenni
for always being happy for my happiness, and for supporting my
idea for 52 Lives from day one, even when it sounded a bit weird.

+ My beautiful children, Abbey, Max and Joseph – you have so much
kindness inside you (even though I know you forget sometimes!) and
I love you more than anything. I promise to turn my computer off
and play more now.

+ And finally to Greig, my love and my best friend who inspired so
many parts of this book. You exude the kind of love, kindness
and warmth that instantly lifts everyone around you. It comes so
naturally to you that you seem to have no awareness of just how
big an impact you have on every person you meet. Every single day
we're together you help me feel loved, capable, beautiful and kind
– even on the days that I'm none of those things.

224